COMPLETE VOLUMETRICS DIET COOKBOOK RECIPES

Discovering the Joy of Cooking
with Complete Volumetrics Diet
Recipes for beginners

Norval Ernser

Copyright

No part of this publication may be reproduced, distributed, or transmitted in any form or by any means, including photocopying, recording, or other electronic or mechanical methods, without the prior written permission of the publisher, except in the case of brief quotations embodied in critical reviews and certain other noncommercial uses permitted by copyright law.

Table of contents

Introduction

Once upon a time, in a quiet little town, there lived a woman named Emily who was on a quest for a healthier lifestyle. She had heard whispers about a magical book called the "Complete Volumetrics Diet Cookbook Recipes," rumored to contain the secrets to crafting delicious and nutritious meals that could transform one's well-being.

Emily, intrigued by the promise of this enchanted cookbook, decided to seek it out. Guided by the excitement of a potential culinary adventure, she ventured to the town's quaint bookstore.

As Emily approached the counter, she inquired about the legendary cookbook. Ms. Harper, a keeper of knowledge and wisdom, smiled knowingly. She reached behind the counter and produced the very book Emily sought – "Complete Volumetrics Diet Cookbook Recipes."

The book's cover gleamed with vibrant of mouthwatering dishes, and the title beckoned to

Emily like a beacon of culinary enlightenment. Little did she know that within those pages, a transformative journey awaited her.

Without hesitation, Emily delved into the cookbook, absorbing its wisdom through the carefully crafted titles and tantalizing recipe descriptions. As if by magic, she felt a newfound understanding of how to prepare meals that were not only delicious but also aligned with the principles of the Volumetrics Diet.

The first chapter, **"UNDERSTANDING VOLUMETRICS DIET,"** revealed the secrets behind the diet's principles. Emily learned about the magic of high-volume, low-calorie foods and how they could be the key to a more satisfying and healthful way of eating.

The subsequent chapters, each with its own captivating title, guided Emily through the art of crafting balanced and flavorful meals. **"ESSENTIAL TOOLS AND INGREDIENTS"** unveiled the secrets of a well-equipped kitchen. "Vibrant Lunch Options" and "Flavorful Dinner

Favorites" inspired her to create culinary masterpieces that celebrated both nutrition and taste.

Emily's kitchen came alive with the aromas of **"BREAKFAST DELIGHTS"** like energizing smoothies and protein-packed bowls. She effortlessly whipped up **"SMART SNACKS AND DESSERTS"** that satisfied her cravings without compromising her commitment to health.

As Emily continued her culinary journey, she discovered the practical aspects of crafting simple meal plans tailored to her lifestyle. The cookbook's guidance on balancing macros within the voluminous principles became her compass, leading her towards meals that not only nourished her body but also brought joy to her taste buds.

Word of Emily's newfound culinary prowess spread throughout the town. Friends and neighbors marveled at the delectable and healthful creations that emerged from her kitchen, all thanks to the magical wisdom contained within the "Complete Volumetrics Diet Cookbook Recipes."

In the end, Emily not only achieved her goal of a healthier lifestyle but also became a beacon of inspiration for others in the town. The enchanted cookbook had not just equipped her with recipes; it had empowered her to embrace a lifestyle where each meal was a celebration of well-being.

And so, the story of Emily and the magical cookbook spread far and wide, inspiring others to embark on their own culinary adventures, armed with the wisdom of the "Complete Volumetrics Diet Cookbook Recipes." The little town blossomed into a haven of health and happiness, all thanks to the transformative magic hidden within the pages of a simple yet extraordinary cookbook.

Chapter 1: Understanding Volumetrics Diet

Welcome to the world of Volumetrics, a revolutionary approach to weight loss and overall well-being. In this chapter, we'll delve into the core concepts of the Volumetrics Diet, introducing you to its principles and guiding you on the journey to a healthier lifestyle. Learn how the philosophy of volumetrics emphasizes the importance of eating foods that provide high volume with low calorie density, allowing you to enjoy satisfying portions while achieving your weight loss goals.

The Science Behind Volumetrics

Uncover the science that makes Volumetrics an effective and sustainable dietary strategy. Explore how the focus on nutrient-rich, water-dense foods can help you feel fuller for longer, leading to reduced calorie intake without sacrificing satiety.

We'll break down the research and principles behind the Volumetrics Diet, giving you the knowledge to make informed choices for your health.

Benefits of Volumetrics for Weight Loss

Discover the numerous benefits that embracing the Volumetrics lifestyle can bring to your weight loss journey. From improved portion control and increased satisfaction to long-term sustainability, we'll explore how this approach goes beyond conventional dieting, fostering a positive relationship with food and promoting lasting results.

Getting Started with the Volumetrics Lifestyle

Ready to embark on your Volumetrics journey? This section provides practical tips and guidance on incorporating the Volumetrics principles into your daily life. From mindful eating practices to strategic food choices, you'll gain insights into making the Volumetrics Diet a seamless and enjoyable part of your lifestyle. Get ready to take the first steps towards a healthier, happier you.

In the next chapter, we'll guide you through the essential tools and ingredients needed to create delicious and nutritious meals that align with the Volumetrics philosophy. Get ready to transform the way you eat and experience the positive impact of the Volumetrics Diet on your overall well-being.

Introduction to Volumetrics

Welcome to the transformative world of Volumetrics, a groundbreaking approach to achieving your weight loss goals and fostering a healthier, happier lifestyle. In this chapter, we will unravel the foundational principles of the Volumetrics Diet, offering you a comprehensive introduction to this innovative and sustainable way of eating.

The Volumetrics Diet is not just a temporary solution; it's a holistic lifestyle that focuses on the quality and quantity of the foods you consume. At its core, Volumetrics encourages you to prioritize foods that provide high volume with low calorie density. This means you can enjoy larger portions of nutrient-dense foods, promoting a sense of fullness and satisfaction without the burden of excessive calories.

The Science Behind Volumetrics

To truly understand the power of Volumetrics, it's essential to explore the scientific underpinnings that make this approach so effective. We'll delve into the research-backed principles that emphasize the importance of water content, fiber, and overall nutritional value in the foods you choose. Learn how these elements contribute to a sense of satiety, allowing you to naturally control your caloric intake.

By adopting the Volumetrics philosophy, you're not just embarking on a diet; you're embracing a lifestyle rooted in evidence-based nutritional science. This chapter will empower you with knowledge, enabling you to make informed choices about the foods you consume and how they impact your overall well-being.

Benefits of Volumetrics for Weight Loss

Embarking on the Volumetrics journey offers a multitude of benefits beyond just shedding pounds. We'll explore how this approach helps you develop sustainable habits, making weight loss not only achievable but maintainable in the long run. From improved energy levels to enhanced mood, discover the holistic advantages of embracing the Volumetrics lifestyle.

Say goodbye to restrictive diets that leave you hungry and dissatisfied. With Volumetrics, you can enjoy a variety of flavorful, filling foods while achieving and maintaining a healthy weight. This chapter will illuminate the pathway to a more balanced and fulfilling relationship with food.

Getting Started with the Volumetrics Lifestyle

Now that you're acquainted with the fundamentals, it's time to take practical steps towards integrating Volumetrics into your daily life. Learn about mindful eating practices, strategic food choices, and simple lifestyle adjustments that will set you on the path to success. This section is your guide to initiating positive changes and experiencing the benefits of the Volumetrics Diet firsthand.

In the upcoming chapters, we will delve deeper into essential tools, ingredients, and mouthwatering recipes that align with the Volumetrics principles. Get ready to embark on a journey of transformation, where health and happiness intersect through the lens of Volumetrics.

The Science Behind Volumetrics

Now, let's delve into the scientific foundations that make the Volumetrics Diet an evidence-based and effective approach to achieving sustainable weight loss and promoting overall well-being.

At the heart of Volumetrics is a profound understanding of how our bodies interact with food and respond to different types of nutrients. The principles are rooted in research that highlights the significance of two key factors: water content and calorie density.

Water Content: One of the cornerstones of Volumetrics is the emphasis on foods with high water content. Many fruits and vegetables, for example, are rich in water, contributing to their low calorie density. The presence of water not only adds volume to the food but also enhances its weight, creating a sense of fullness without a surplus of calories. This means you can enjoy larger portions of these foods, providing satisfaction while supporting your weight loss goals.

Calorie Density: Calorie density refers to the number of calories in a given volume of food. Volumetrics encourages the consumption of foods with low calorie density, allowing you to eat more while still maintaining a calorie deficit. By focusing on nutrient-dense options, you not only supply your body with essential vitamins and minerals but also naturally regulate your caloric intake. This strategic approach enables you to feel satiated, making it easier to adhere to your dietary goals.

Research studies consistently demonstrate that diets rich in low-calorie-dense foods, particularly fruits and vegetables, contribute to weight loss and improved overall health. Understanding the science behind Volumetrics empowers you to make informed choices, transforming the way you approach meals and snacks.

As you incorporate Volumetrics into your lifestyle, keep in mind that the science is not just about shedding pounds. It's about fostering a sustainable and enjoyable relationship with food that supports your long-term health and well-being. In the next section, we'll explore the specific benefits of adopting the Volumetrics lifestyle, shedding light on how this approach goes beyond traditional diets to enhance various aspects of your life.

Benefits of Volumetrics for Weight Loss

Embarking on the Volumetrics journey extends beyond mere weight loss; it's a holistic approach that offers a myriad of benefits for your overall well-being. Let's explore how adopting the Volumetrics lifestyle can positively impact various facets of your health.

1. Sustainable Weight Loss: The primary goal of Volumetrics is to help you shed excess weight in a sustainable and maintainable way. By focusing on foods with high water content and low calorie density, you can create a calorie deficit without the discomfort of restrictive diets. This approach not only facilitates weight loss but also encourages a long-term commitment to healthier eating habits.

2. Increased Satiety: Volumetrics isn't about deprivation; it's about satisfaction. The emphasis on nutrient-dense, filling foods means you can enjoy larger portions without consuming excessive calories. This leads to increased satiety, making it easier to adhere to your dietary goals without constantly feeling hungry or deprived.

3. Improved Nutrient Intake: Volumetrics places a spotlight on foods rich in essential nutrients such as vitamins, minerals, and antioxidants. By incorporating a variety of fruits, vegetables, and whole grains into your diet, you not only support weight loss but also provide your body with the nutrients it needs for optimal functioning and overall health.

4. Enhanced Energy Levels: Unlike crash diets that may leave you feeling fatigued, the balanced and nutritious nature of the Volumetrics Diet ensures that your body receives the energy it requires. Experience a sustained energy boost throughout the day, promoting overall vitality and well-being.

5. Positive Mood and Mental Well-Being: The connection between diet and mental health is well-established, and Volumetrics is no exception. A diet rich in nutrient-dense foods has been linked to improved mood and cognitive function. By nourishing your body with the right foods, you not only support your physical health but also contribute to a positive mental state.

6. Long-Term Lifestyle Change: Volumetrics isn't a quick fix; it's a lifestyle change. The sustainable and flexible nature of this approach means you can seamlessly integrate it into your daily life. Say goodbye to the cycle of yo-yo dieting, and hello to a balanced and enjoyable way of eating that lasts.

As we continue our exploration into the Volumetrics Diet, the next section will guide you on practical steps to initiate this lifestyle change. Discover how to seamlessly incorporate Volumetrics into your daily routine, setting the stage for a healthier and happier you.

Getting Started with the Volumetrics Lifestyle

Now that you've gained insight into the science and benefits of the Volumetrics Diet, it's time to take practical steps towards embracing this transformative lifestyle. This section will guide you through the essential aspects of initiating the Volumetrics approach into your daily routine, making it a seamless and enjoyable part of your life.

Mindful Eating Practices:

Begin your Volumetrics journey by cultivating mindful eating habits. Pay attention to your body's hunger and fullness cues. Slow down during meals, savoring each bite. By being present and attentive, you can develop a deeper connection with your food and cultivate a more satisfying eating experience.

Strategic Food Choices:

Understanding the principles of Volumetrics empowers you to make strategic food choices. Opt for foods with high water content, such as fruits and vegetables, to maximize volume without excess calories. Choose lean proteins, whole grains, and healthy fats to create balanced and nutritious meals. The goal is to enjoy a variety of foods that align with Volumetrics principles.

Smart Snacking:

Snacking can be a part of a healthy Volumetrics lifestyle. Discover smart snack options that keep you energized between meals without derailing your progress. Explore the world of nutrient-dense snacks, incorporating fruits, vegetables, and protein-rich choices to maintain satiety throughout the day.

Hydration Matters:

Water is a fundamental component of the Volumetrics approach. Stay well-hydrated to support the filling effect of water-rich foods and promote overall health. Hydration is a simple yet powerful tool to complement your dietary efforts and enhance the effectiveness of the Volumetrics lifestyle.

Meal Planning for Success:

Efficient meal planning is a key element of successfully adopting the Volumetrics Diet. Learn how to create balanced and satisfying meals that align with your preferences and lifestyle. Discover easy-to-implement strategies for weekly meal planning, ensuring that you have nutritious options readily available and reducing the likelihood of making less healthy choices.

Tailoring Volumetrics to Your Lifestyle:

Recognize that the Volumetrics Diet is adaptable to different lifestyles. Whether you have a busy schedule, dietary preferences, or specific health considerations, this section will guide you in tailoring the Volumetrics principles to suit your individual needs. Flexibility is a strength of the Volumetrics lifestyle, making it accessible to a diverse range of individuals.

By incorporating these practical steps into your daily routine, you'll be well on your way to embracing the Volumetrics lifestyle. In the upcoming chapters, we will dive deeper into the tools and ingredients essential for creating delicious and nutritious meals that align with the Volumetrics philosophy. Get ready to embark on a journey where health and happiness converge through the lens of Volumetrics.

Chapter 2: Essential Tools and Ingredients

Now that you're acquainted with the foundational principles of the Volumetrics Diet, it's time to equip yourself with the essential tools and ingredients that will turn your kitchen into a hub of nutritious and flavorful creations. This chapter will guide you through the key elements necessary to embark on your Volumetrics journey successfully.

Kitchen Must-Haves for Volumetrics Cooking:

Discover the essential tools that will make preparing Volumetrics-inspired meals a breeze. From kitchen gadgets that streamline meal prep to cookware that enhances the flavors of your dishes, this section will outline the must-have items that will set you up for success in the Volumetrics kitchen.

Key Ingredients for Flavorful and Nutrient-Rich Meals:

Explore the palette of ingredients that form the foundation of Volumetrics cooking. From vibrant fruits and vegetables to lean proteins and whole grains, we'll delve into the nutritional powerhouses that will not only support your weight loss goals but also contribute to overall well-being. Learn how to create a well-stocked kitchen that enables you to whip up delicious and satisfying meals at a moment's notice.

Smart Grocery Shopping for Volumetrics Success:

Navigate the aisles with confidence as we guide you through the art of smart grocery shopping for the Volumetrics lifestyle. Learn to decipher food labels, choose fresh and seasonal produce, and make informed decisions about the foods you bring into your home. Transform your grocery trips into opportunities to nourish your body and align with the principles of the Volumetrics Diet.

Armed with the knowledge of essential tools and ingredients, you'll be ready to transform your kitchen into a space where health-conscious and delicious meals come together effortlessly. In the upcoming chapters, we'll delve into mouthwatering recipes specifically crafted for the Volumetrics lifestyle. Get ready to explore a world of flavors that nourish both your body and your taste buds.

Kitchen Must-Haves for Volumetrics Cooking

Creating delicious and nutritious meals in line with the Volumetrics Diet requires a well-equipped kitchen. Let's explore the essential tools that will streamline your cooking process and make your culinary adventures a joy.

1. High-Quality Blender:

Invest in a powerful blender to craft satisfying and nutrient-packed smoothies, soups, and sauces. A blender is a versatile tool that allows you to incorporate a variety of fruits, vegetables, and liquids, creating meals with the desired volume and flavor.

2. Precision Measuring Tools:

Accurate portion control is a key aspect of Volumetrics. Equip your kitchen with measuring cups and spoons to ensure you're using the right amounts of ingredients. This precision will help you maintain the balance of flavors and nutritional content in your meals.

3. Steam Basket:

Steaming is an excellent cooking method in the Volumetrics kitchen. A steam basket preserves the nutritional value of vegetables while enhancing their natural flavors. Use this tool to prepare crisp and vibrant veggies that contribute to the high-volume, low-calorie nature of Volumetrics meals.

4. Non-Stick Cookware:

Invest in high-quality non-stick cookware to minimize the need for excessive fats and oils in your cooking. This ensures that your meals are not only flavorful but also aligned with the Volumetrics philosophy of reducing calorie density while maximizing volume.

5. Food Scale:

A food scale is a handy tool for precise measurements, particularly when portion control is crucial. Use it to accurately measure ingredients and track your portions, aiding you in maintaining the balance of your Volumetrics meals.

6. Spiralizer:

For a creative twist on low-calorie, high-volume meals, a spiralizer is a fantastic addition. Transform vegetables like zucchini and carrots into noodle-like strands, adding variety and texture to your dishes without compromising on nutrition.

7. Herb and Spice Collection:

Flavor is paramount in Volumetrics cooking, and herbs and spices play a crucial role in achieving delicious meals without excess calories. Build a diverse collection of herbs and spices to elevate the taste of your dishes without relying on heavy sauces or dressings.

8. Storage Containers:

Prepare Volumetrics meals in batches and store them in portion-sized containers. This not only simplifies meal planning but also ensures that you have nutritious options readily available, reducing the temptation to opt for less healthy alternatives.

By incorporating these kitchen must-haves, you'll be well-equipped to embark on your Volumetrics cooking journey. In the next section, we'll explore the key ingredients that form the foundation of flavorful and nutrient-rich Volumetrics meals. Get ready to fill your kitchen with the tools that will turn your culinary aspirations into delicious and healthful realities.

Key Ingredients for Flavorful and Nutrient-Rich Meals

Now that your kitchen is equipped with essential tools, let's dive into the key ingredients that form the foundation of delectable and nutrient-rich meals in line with the Volumetrics Diet. These ingredients are not only flavorful but also packed with the nutrients your body needs for optimal health.

1. Vibrant Fruits:

Incorporate a variety of fresh, seasonal fruits into your Volumetrics repertoire. Berries, citrus fruits, apples, and melons are not only delicious but also rich in vitamins, minerals, and antioxidants. Use them in smoothies, salads, and desserts to add natural sweetness and volume to your meals.

2. Colorful Vegetables:

Load up on colorful vegetables to enhance the visual appeal and nutritional content of your dishes. Leafy greens, bell peppers, tomatoes, broccoli, and carrots are excellent choices. These vegetables are low in calories and high in fiber, contributing to the filling nature of Volumetrics meals.

3. Lean Proteins:

Incorporate lean protein sources to support muscle health and keep you feeling satisfied. Skinless poultry, lean cuts of beef or pork, fish, tofu, and legumes are excellent choices. Proteins contribute to the overall volume of your meals while providing essential nutrients.

4. Whole Grains:

Opt for whole grains to add fiber and complexity to your Volumetrics meals. Quinoa, brown rice, oats, and whole wheat products are nutritious choices that contribute to sustained energy levels and a feeling of fullness.

5. Healthy Fats:

Include sources of healthy fats to add richness and flavor to your meals without compromising on nutrition. Avocado, nuts, seeds, and olive oil are great options. These fats contribute to satiety and support the absorption of fat-soluble vitamins.

6. Greek Yogurt and Low-Fat Dairy:

Dairy products like Greek yogurt and low-fat options are excellent sources of protein and calcium. They add creaminess to your recipes without excess calories, making them valuable additions to Volumetrics-friendly dishes.

7. Herbs and Spices:

Elevate the taste of your meals with a diverse collection of herbs and spices. Fresh herbs like basil, cilantro, and mint, along with spices such as cumin, turmeric, and paprika, can add depth and flavor without the need for excessive salt or high-calorie sauces.

8. Beans and Legumes:

Beans and legumes are nutrient-dense, high-fiber ingredients that contribute to the satisfying nature of Volumetrics meals. Incorporate lentils, chickpeas, black beans, and other legumes into soups, salads, and main dishes.

By keeping your kitchen stocked with these key ingredients, you'll have the building blocks for crafting flavorful and nutrient-packed meals in line with the Volumetrics philosophy. In the next section, we'll explore the art of smart grocery shopping to ensure you consistently have these ingredients on hand. Get ready to embark on a journey of culinary creativity and nourishment.

Smart Grocery Shopping for Volumetrics Success

Mastering the art of smart grocery shopping is a fundamental aspect of successfully integrating the Volumetrics Diet into your lifestyle. Let's explore practical strategies and tips to ensure your grocery trips align with the principles of Volumetrics, keeping your kitchen stocked with the essentials for delicious and healthful meals.

1. Plan Your Meals in Advance:

Before heading to the grocery store, plan your meals for the week. This not only helps you create a comprehensive shopping list but also prevents impulse purchases. Focus on incorporating a variety of colorful fruits, vegetables, lean proteins, whole grains, and healthy fats into your meal plans.

2. Prioritize Fresh Produce:

The majority of your grocery cart should be filled with fresh produce. Choose a rainbow of fruits and vegetables, opting for seasonal and locally sourced options when possible. These nutrient-dense foods will form the backbone of your Volumetrics meals, providing essential vitamins, minerals, and fiber.

3. Explore the Perimeter:

Navigate the grocery store's perimeter, where you'll find fresh produce, lean proteins, dairy, and whole grains. This strategy helps you avoid the tempting, calorie-dense aisles filled with processed and packaged foods. The perimeter typically houses the whole, unprocessed ingredients essential for Volumetrics cooking.

4. Read Labels Mindfully:

When venturing into the central aisles, be mindful of food labels. Choose whole, minimally processed foods and be wary of items high in added sugars, sodium, and unhealthy fats. The goal is to select nutrient-dense options that contribute to the satisfying and healthful nature of Volumetrics meals.

5. Buy in Bulk Smartly:

Consider purchasing staple items like whole grains, legumes, and nuts in bulk. This not only reduces packaging waste but also saves money in the long run. Bulk purchases ensure you have a consistent supply of these key ingredients for crafting voluminous and nutritious meals.

6. Stock Up on Frozen Produce:

Frozen fruits and vegetables are convenient, budget-friendly alternatives to fresh produce, especially when certain items are out of season. Frozen options retain their nutritional value and can be a valuable resource for creating quick and easy Volumetrics meals.

7. Choose Lean Proteins:

Prioritize lean protein sources such as poultry, fish, tofu, and legumes. Opt for cuts of meat with minimal visible fat and explore plant-based protein options to add variety to your diet. These proteins contribute to the volume of your meals while supporting your overall health goals.

8. Don't Forget Healthy Fats:

Include sources of healthy fats, such as avocados, nuts, seeds, and olive oil, in your shopping list.

These ingredients add richness and flavor to your meals without compromising the principles of the Volumetrics Diet. They contribute to satiety and enhance the overall eating experience.

Armed with these smart grocery shopping strategies, you'll be well-prepared to fill your kitchen with the key ingredients needed for Volumetrics success. In the following chapters, we'll translate these ingredients into mouthwatering recipes that make embracing the Volumetrics lifestyle both delightful and nourishing. Get ready to embark on a culinary journey that prioritizes both health and flavor.

Chapter 3: Breakfast Delights

Welcome to the heart of your day, where we transform breakfast into a delightful and nourishing experience that aligns seamlessly with the Volumetrics Diet. In this chapter, we'll explore a variety of morning options designed to kickstart your day with flavor, energy, and the satisfying principles of volumetrics.

Energizing Morning Smoothies:

Start your day with a burst of nutrients by embracing energizing morning smoothies. These customizable concoctions allow you to blend a variety of fruits, vegetables, lean proteins, and healthy fats. We'll explore delicious combinations that not only tantalize your taste buds but also provide the volume and nutrition needed to keep you full and focused throughout the morning.

Wholesome Oat-Based Creations:

Oats are a Volumetrics superstar, offering a hearty and fiber-rich base for a myriad of breakfast creations. Dive into the world of wholesome oat-based delights, from comforting bowls of oatmeal topped with fresh fruits and nuts to creative overnight oats that simplify your morning routine. Discover how oats can become the canvas for a satisfying and nutritious breakfast.

Protein-Packed Breakfast Bowls:

Craft protein-packed breakfast bowls that are both filling and flavorful. Explore savory options with eggs, vegetables, and lean proteins or indulge in sweet variations featuring Greek yogurt, berries, and granola. These breakfast bowls offer a versatile and customizable way to create meals that align with the Volumetrics principles, ensuring a satiating start to your day.

As we embark on this journey through breakfast delights, remember that each recipe is not only designed to tantalize your taste buds but also to set the tone for a day of balanced and fulfilling eating.

Get ready to revolutionize your mornings with Volumetrics-inspired breakfasts that nourish both your body and soul.

Energizing Morning Smoothies

Rise and shine with the vibrant and invigorating world of energizing morning smoothies. These delicious concoctions are not just a feast for your taste buds but also a powerhouse of nutrients, perfectly aligned with the principles of the Volumetrics Diet. Let's explore a variety of recipes that will kickstart your day with vitality and satisfaction.

1. Berry Blast Smoothie:
Blend together a symphony of antioxidant-rich berries, such as blueberries, strawberries, and raspberries, with a base of low-fat Greek yogurt. Add a handful of spinach for an extra nutrient boost without compromising the delightful taste. The

result is a refreshing and energizing smoothie that's as visually appealing as it is nutritious.

2. Green Goddess Delight:

Unleash the power of greens with a Green Goddess smoothie. Combine spinach or kale with a banana, pineapple chunks, and a splash of coconut water. The combination of leafy greens and tropical fruits creates a revitalizing smoothie that's not only good for your taste buds but also supports your body with essential vitamins and minerals.

3. Protein-Packed Peanut Butter Bliss:

For a satisfying and protein-rich option, blend together a banana, a scoop of peanut butter, low-fat milk or a dairy-free alternative, and a dash of cinnamon. The natural sweetness of the banana combined with the richness of peanut butter creates a creamy and indulgent smoothie that will keep you fueled and satisfied.

4. Tropical Paradise Smoothie:

Transport yourself to a tropical paradise with a blend of mango, pineapple, and coconut milk. Add a scoop of protein powder or Greek yogurt for an extra boost of protein. The tropical flavors combined with the smooth texture make this smoothie a delightful way to start your day with a touch of paradise.

5. Chia Berry Powerhouse:

Incorporate the nutritional powerhouse, chia seeds, into your morning routine with a Chia Berry smoothie. Blend together mixed berries, almond milk, and a tablespoon of chia seeds. The chia seeds add a dose of omega-3 fatty acids and contribute to the satisfying volume of the smoothie.

Remember, the beauty of morning smoothies lies not only in their taste but in their versatility. Feel free to customize these recipes based on your preferences and the ingredients you have on hand. With energizing morning smoothies, you'll set a vibrant tone for your day while embracing the fulfilling principles of the Volumetrics Diet. Get ready to sip your way to a nourishing morning!

Wholesome Oat-Based Creations

Breakfast becomes a hearty affair with the introduction of wholesome oat-based creations. Oats, a Volumetrics staple, take center stage in these satisfying and nutritious morning options. Let's explore a variety of recipes that transform oats into delightful breakfasts, providing both sustenance and flavor in line with the principles of the Volumetrics Diet.

1. Classic Fruit and Nut Oatmeal:
Kickstart your day with a classic bowl of oatmeal adorned with a medley of fresh fruits and a sprinkle of nuts. Choose from toppings like sliced bananas, berries, and a handful of almonds or walnuts. The combination of fiber-rich oats and nutrient-dense fruits creates a filling and delicious breakfast that fuels your morning.

2. Overnight Chia Oats:
Simplify your mornings with Overnight Chia Oats, a convenient and nutritious option. Combine oats,

chia seeds, and your choice of milk or yogurt in a jar, and let it sit in the refrigerator overnight. Wake up to a creamy and textured breakfast that can be personalized with toppings like sliced fruits, nuts, or a drizzle of honey.

3. Savory Spinach and Mushroom Oatmeal:

Explore the savory side of oats with a Spinach and Mushroom Oatmeal. Cook oats with savory broth and stir in sautéed spinach and mushrooms. Top with a sprinkle of Parmesan cheese for a savory and satisfying breakfast that adds variety to your morning routine.

4. Apple Cinnamon Baked Oatmeal:

Infuse your kitchen with the comforting aroma of Apple Cinnamon Baked Oatmeal. Mix oats with diced apples, cinnamon, and a touch of maple syrup, then bake until golden brown. This warm and flavorful dish is perfect for a cozy breakfast that feels indulgent yet aligns with the nutritious principles of Volumetrics.

5. Yogurt Parfait with Oat Clusters:

Layer your morning with a Yogurt Parfait featuring crunchy oat clusters. Combine oats, nuts, and a hint of honey, then bake to create clusters that add a satisfying crunch to your parfait. Alternate layers of yogurt with these oat clusters and fresh berries for a visually appealing and delightful breakfast.

These wholesome oat-based creations not only provide a delicious start to your day but also leverage the voluminous nature of oats to keep you satisfied until your next meal. Customize these recipes to suit your taste preferences and dietary needs, and embrace the fulfilling potential of oats in your morning routine. Get ready to enjoy breakfast in a way that nourishes both your body and your taste buds!

Protein-Packed Breakfast Bowls

Elevate your mornings with the robust and filling appeal of Protein-Packed Breakfast Bowls. These breakfast creations are designed to not only tantalize your taste buds but also provide a satisfying and protein-rich foundation for your day, aligning perfectly with the principles of the Volumetrics Diet. Let's explore a variety of recipes that infuse your mornings with both flavor and nourishment.

1. Veggie-Packed Egg White Scramble:
Start your day with a protein boost by crafting a Veggie-Packed Egg White Scramble. Whisk together egg whites and sauté them with an assortment of colorful vegetables such as bell peppers, spinach, and tomatoes. Top with a sprinkle of feta cheese for a savory and nutrient-rich breakfast bowl.

2. Greek Yogurt and Berry Bliss:
Indulge in a delightful blend of protein and sweetness with a Greek Yogurt and Berry Bliss bowl. Layer high-protein Greek yogurt with a variety of fresh berries, granola, and a drizzle of honey. This combination not only satisfies your sweet cravings but also provides a hearty and protein-packed start to your day.

3. Smoked Salmon and Avocado Quinoa Bowl:

Create an elegant and protein-rich breakfast with a Smoked Salmon and Avocado Quinoa Bowl. Combine flaked smoked salmon, creamy avocado slices, and cooked quinoa for a bowl that's not only rich in omega-3 fatty acids but also incredibly satisfying.

4. Plant-Powered Protein Bowl:

For a plant-based protein option, assemble a Plant-Powered Protein Bowl. Combine ingredients like cooked lentils, chickpeas, quinoa, and a variety of vegetables. Drizzle with a tahini dressing for added flavor and creaminess. This bowl showcases the versatility of plant-based proteins for a hearty and nutritious morning meal.

5. Nutty Banana Protein Smoothie Bowl:

Blend together a Nutty Banana Protein Smoothie Bowl that combines the goodness of protein-rich Greek yogurt, a ripe banana, and a scoop of your favorite protein powder. Top with nuts, seeds, and sliced banana for a delightful and crunchy texture that makes every bite a protein-packed delight.

These Protein-Packed Breakfast Bowls not only cater to your taste preferences but also ensure that you start your day with a satisfying and nutrient-dense meal. Experiment with different ingredients, textures, and flavors to find the perfect protein bowl that suits your morning routine. With these recipes, you'll embrace a breakfast that not only fuels your day but also aligns with the fulfilling principles of the Volumetrics Diet. Get ready to savor every protein-packed bite!

Chapter 4: Vibrant Lunch Options

Lunchtime is an opportunity to refuel and recharge, and with the Volumetrics Diet, it's also a chance to indulge in vibrant and satisfying meals that support your health and well-being. In this chapter, we'll explore a spectrum of colorful and nutrient-dense lunch options that bring excitement to your midday break while adhering to the principles of the Volumetrics Diet.

Fresh and Flavorful Salad Creations:

Salads are more than just a side dish; they can be the star of your lunch, providing a plethora of nutrients and textures. Let's delve into creative salad recipes that go beyond the typical greens, incorporating a variety of vegetables, proteins, and dressings to create a satisfying and vibrant lunch experience.

Wholesome Grain-Based Bowls:

Grain-based bowls offer a hearty and nourishing lunch option that combines whole grains with an array of vegetables, proteins, and flavorful dressings. Explore diverse combinations that bring together ingredients like quinoa, brown rice, or farro with vibrant vegetables and lean proteins to create bowls that are both filling and visually appealing.

Energizing Wrap and Roll Creations:

Elevate your lunch with energizing wrap and roll creations that bring together a variety of ingredients in a convenient and portable format. From veggie wraps with hummus to protein-packed roll-ups, these options provide a satisfying and flavorful way to enjoy a balanced lunch that aligns with the Volumetrics principles.

Hearty Soup and Stew Varieties:

Warm up your lunchtime with hearty soup and stew varieties that not only comfort your soul but also provide a voluminous and nutrient-rich meal. From vegetable-packed minestrone to protein-rich chicken stew, these recipes will keep you full and satisfied throughout the afternoon, showcasing the versatility of soups in Volumetrics dining.

Bountiful Buddha Bowls:

Buddha bowls are a feast for the eyes and the palate, offering a balanced combination of grains, proteins, and an assortment of colorful vegetables. Explore the art of crafting bountiful Buddha bowls that cater to your taste preferences while adhering to the filling principles of the Volumetrics Diet.

Get ready to transform your lunchtime routine with these vibrant and satisfying options. Whether you prefer a refreshing salad, a wholesome grain bowl, a convenient wrap, a comforting soup, or a colorful Buddha bowl, these recipes will bring joy and nourishment to your midday break. Embrace the variety, colors, and flavors that Volumetrics has to offer in your lunchtime endeavors!

Fresh and Filling Salads

Lunchtime takes on a new level of excitement with fresh and filling salads that go beyond the ordinary. Embrace a spectrum of flavors, textures, and nutrients as we explore creative salad recipes designed to satisfy your taste buds and keep you energized throughout the day, all while adhering to the principles of the Volumetrics Diet.

1. Mediterranean Quinoa Salad:

Transport your taste buds to the Mediterranean with a Quinoa Salad that combines fluffy quinoa with cherry tomatoes, cucumber, olives, and feta cheese. Drizzle with a lemon-oregano dressing to create a refreshing and protein-packed salad that's both vibrant and satisfying.

2. Southwest Chicken and Avocado Salad:

Bring a touch of the Southwest to your lunch with a Chicken and Avocado Salad. Grill or roast chicken breast, then toss it with a mix of crisp lettuce, black beans, corn, cherry tomatoes, and creamy avocado. Top with a zesty lime-cilantro dressing for a colorful and protein-rich salad.

3. Asian-Inspired Sesame Ginger Salad:

Embark on a culinary journey with an Asian-inspired Sesame Ginger Salad. Combine shredded cabbage, carrots, bell peppers, and edamame. Toss with a flavorful sesame ginger dressing and top with grilled chicken or tofu for a nutrient-packed and satisfying lunch option.

4. Berry and Goat Cheese Spinach Salad:

Indulge in the sweet and savory combination of a Berry and Goat Cheese Spinach Salad. Toss together fresh spinach with a mix of berries, goat cheese crumbles, and candied pecans. Drizzle with a balsamic vinaigrette to create a salad that's both elegant and filling.

5. Roasted Vegetable and Quinoa Bowl:

Roasted vegetables take center stage in this hearty Roasted Vegetable and Quinoa Bowl. Roast a medley of colorful veggies like bell peppers, zucchini, and cherry tomatoes, then mix them with quinoa. Add a sprinkle of feta cheese and a balsamic glaze for a flavorful and nutrient-dense salad bowl.

6. Tuna and Chickpea Salad:

Elevate your protein intake with a Tuna and Chickpea Salad. Mix canned tuna with chickpeas, cherry tomatoes, cucumber, and red onion. Drizzle with a lemon-tahini dressing for a satisfying and protein-packed salad that keeps you full and fueled.

These fresh and filling salads not only showcase the vibrant colors of a variety of ingredients but also deliver a satisfying and nutritious lunch experience. Feel free to customize these recipes based on your preferences, and embrace the joy of incorporating vibrant salads into your lunchtime routine. With these options, you'll discover that salads can be both a delightful and substantial choice, aligning perfectly with the principles of the Volumetrics Diet.

Hearty Soups for Satisfying Lunches

Warm up your lunchtime with a delightful array of hearty soups that not only comfort your soul but also provide a nourishing and satisfying meal. These recipes showcase the versatility of soups in the Volumetrics dining experience, offering a comforting yet filling option for your midday break.

1. Vegetable and Lentil Minestrone:
Savor the goodness of a Vegetable and Lentil Minestrone that brings together a medley of colorful vegetables, hearty lentils, and aromatic herbs. This nutritious and filling soup is a perfect blend of flavors that will leave you satisfied and energized for the rest of the day.

2. Chicken and Wild Rice Soup:
Indulge in the warmth of a classic Chicken and Wild Rice Soup that combines tender chicken, wild rice, and a variety of vegetables in a rich and flavorful broth. This hearty soup provides a comforting lunch option that's both filling and wholesome.

3. Tomato Basil Quinoa Soup:

Elevate the classic tomato soup with the addition of quinoa and fresh basil. The Tomato Basil Quinoa Soup is a delightful twist on a familiar favorite, offering a satisfying blend of textures and flavors that make it a perfect choice for a wholesome and voluminous lunch.

4. Spicy Black Bean and Vegetable Chili:

Kick up the heat with a Spicy Black Bean and Vegetable Chili. This protein-packed soup combines black beans, vibrant vegetables, and bold spices for a chili that's not only satisfying but also delivers a nutritional punch. Top it with a dollop of Greek yogurt and fresh cilantro for added richness.

5. Butternut Squash and Apple Bisque:

Embrace the cozy flavors of fall with a Butternut Squash and Apple Bisque. This velvety soup combines the natural sweetness of butternut squash with the tartness of apples, creating a delightful and filling bisque that's perfect for a satisfying lunch.

6. Lentil and Spinach Stew:

Experience the heartiness of a Lentil and Spinach Stew that marries protein-packed lentils with nutrient-dense spinach. Infused with aromatic spices, this stew provides a satisfying and flavorful lunch option that's as nourishing as it is delicious.

These hearty soups not only warm your soul but also keep you full and content throughout the afternoon. Feel free to experiment with ingredients, adjust spice levels, and customize these recipes to suit your taste preferences. With these options, you'll discover the joy of incorporating hearty soups into your lunchtime routine while staying true to the principles of the Volumetrics Diet.

Quick and Easy Lunch Wraps

Lunchtime just got a whole lot more exciting with quick and easy lunch wraps that not only cater to your on-the-go lifestyle but also embrace the vibrant and satisfying principles of the Volumetrics Diet. Let's explore a variety of creative wrap recipes that bring together diverse flavors, textures, and nutrients for a lunch that's both convenient and fulfilling.

1. Veggie Hummus Wrap:

Wrap up a medley of colorful vegetables, such as bell peppers, cucumber, carrots, and spinach, with a generous spread of hummus. Add a sprinkle of feta cheese for a creamy touch. This Veggie Hummus Wrap is not only quick to assemble but also a delightful explosion of flavors and textures.

2. Turkey and Avocado Wrap:

Combine lean turkey slices with creamy avocado, crisp lettuce, and tomato slices for a protein-packed and refreshing wrap. Drizzle with a light dressing or Greek yogurt for added flavor. This Turkey and Avocado Wrap is a quick and easy lunch option that satisfies both your taste buds and your hunger.

3. Mediterranean Chickpea Wrap:

Create a Mediterranean-inspired wrap by filling a whole-grain tortilla with chickpeas, cherry tomatoes, cucumber, olives, and a drizzle of tzatziki sauce. This flavorful and fiber-rich Mediterranean Chickpea Wrap is a perfect option for a satisfying and quick lunch.

4. Spinach and Feta Turkey Wrap:

Wrap up your lunch in a Spinach and Feta Turkey Wrap that combines lean turkey with fresh spinach, crumbled feta cheese, and a touch of balsamic glaze. This savory and nutritious wrap is a delightful choice for a speedy and satisfying midday meal.

5. BBQ Chicken and Veggie Wrap:

Enjoy the smoky flavors of BBQ chicken in a quick and easy wrap. Combine shredded BBQ chicken with crisp veggies like bell peppers and red onion. Roll it all up in a tortilla for a BBQ Chicken and Veggie Wrap that's both flavorful and filling.

6. Caprese Salad Wrap:

Take the classic Caprese salad to a new level by turning it into a wrap. Fill your tortilla with fresh tomatoes, mozzarella cheese, basil leaves, and a drizzle of balsamic glaze. This Caprese Salad Wrap offers a burst of Mediterranean flavors in a convenient handheld package.

These quick and easy lunch wraps not only cater to your busy schedule but also provide a satisfying and flavorful meal that aligns with the principles of the Volumetrics Diet. Customize these recipes to suit your preferences and enjoy a lunch that's both vibrant and convenient. With these options, you'll discover the joy of embracing quick wraps as a wholesome and filling lunchtime choice.

Chapter 5: Flavorful Dinner Favorites

Dinnertime is an opportunity to indulge in delicious and satisfying meals that bring joy to the table. In this chapter, we'll explore a variety of flavorful dinner favorites that not only cater to your taste buds but also adhere to the principles of the Volumetrics Diet. From wholesome one-pan wonders to inventive takes on classic dishes, these recipes are designed to make your dinners both delicious and fulfilling.

Sizzling Sheet Pan Dinners:

Experience the convenience and vibrancy of sheet pan dinners that bring together a variety of ingredients for a fuss-free and flavorful meal. Let's dive into recipes that showcase the art of one-pan cooking, creating dinners that are not only easy to prepare but also generous in volume and taste.

Nutrient-Rich Grain Bowls:

Grain bowls offer a canvas for creativity, allowing you to combine a variety of nutrient-rich ingredients into a harmonious and satisfying dinner. Explore diverse combinations of grains, proteins, vegetables, and flavorful dressings to create grain bowls that make your dinner both nourishing and delicious.

Inspired Takes on Classic Comforts:

Put a nutritious spin on classic comfort foods with inspired recipes that retain the familiar flavors while aligning with the principles of the Volumetrics Diet. From healthier versions of lasagna to inventive approaches to macaroni and cheese, these dinner favorites provide a comforting yet voluminous dining experience.

Wholesome Stir-Fry Creations:

Stir-fries offer a quick and versatile way to infuse your dinners with a burst of flavors and textures. Explore wholesome stir-fry creations that combine lean proteins, vibrant vegetables, and savory sauces for dinners that are both satisfying and light on calories.

Delectable Seafood Showcases:

Embrace the goodness of the sea with delectable seafood showcases that turn dinner into a culinary adventure. From grilled salmon with citrus glaze to shrimp and vegetable skewers, these recipes bring the freshness and health benefits of seafood to your dinner table.

Savory and Balanced Casseroles:

Casseroles offer a convenient way to create savory and balanced dinners with minimal effort. Discover recipes that transform simple ingredients into hearty and flavorful casseroles, making your dinners both easy to prepare and enjoyable to savor.

Get ready to elevate your dinner experiences with these flavorful favorites. Whether you're a fan of one-pan wonders, nutrient-rich grain bowls, inventive classics, wholesome stir-fries, delightful seafood dishes, or comforting casseroles, these recipes ensure that your dinners are both satisfying and aligned with the principles of the Volumetrics Diet. Let's embark on a journey of flavorful dining that prioritizes both taste and well-being.

Satisfying One-Pan Meals

Experience the ease and delight of satisfying one-pan meals that not only simplify your dinner preparation but also infuse your table with a symphony of flavors. These recipes are a testament to the versatility of one-pan cooking, offering wholesome and voluminous dinners with minimal cleanup.

1. Lemon Herb Roasted Chicken with Vegetables:

Elevate your dinner with a Lemon Herb Roasted Chicken surrounded by a medley of colorful vegetables. The chicken, marinated in zesty lemon and aromatic herbs, roasts to perfection alongside potatoes, carrots, and Brussels sprouts. This one-pan wonder delivers a satisfying and wholesome meal that fills your plate and your senses.

2. Teriyaki Salmon and Vegetable Bake:

Immerse your taste buds in the delightful fusion of flavors with a Teriyaki Salmon and Vegetable Bake. Marinate salmon fillets in a teriyaki glaze, then bake them alongside an array of crisp vegetables like broccoli, bell peppers, and snap peas. This vibrant and nutritious one-pan meal ensures a dinner that's both satisfying and packed with omega-3 fatty acids.

3. Mediterranean Chickpea and Vegetable Skillet:

Embark on a culinary journey to the Mediterranean with a Chickpea and Vegetable Skillet. Sauté chickpeas, cherry tomatoes, artichoke hearts, and spinach in a blend of olive oil, garlic, and Mediterranean spices. This plant-based one-pan meal not only offers a burst of flavors but also showcases the satiating power of wholesome ingredients.

4. Quinoa and Black Bean Fiesta Bowl:

Transform your dinner into a fiesta with a Quinoa and Black Bean Fiesta Bowl. Cook quinoa and black beans with a blend of spices, then top with vibrant ingredients like avocado, tomatoes, and cilantro. This protein-packed and nutrient-rich one-pan meal is both satisfying and visually appealing.

5. Honey Mustard Glazed Pork Chop Sheet Pan:

Indulge in the sweet and savory goodness of a Honey Mustard Glazed Pork Chop Sheet Pan dinner. Marinate pork chops in a honey mustard glaze, then roast them alongside sweet potatoes, green beans, and red onions. This delectable one-pan meal is a harmony of flavors that makes dinner both delightful and wholesome.

6. Ratatouille with Baked Chicken Thighs:

Transport your dinner to the French countryside with a Ratatouille featuring baked chicken thighs. Layer vibrant slices of zucchini, eggplant, and tomatoes alongside succulent chicken thighs for a visually stunning and satisfying one-pan meal that captures the essence of French cuisine.

These satisfying one-pan meals not only simplify your dinner routine but also celebrate the richness and variety of flavors that can be achieved with minimal fuss. Customize these recipes to suit your taste preferences, and savor the joy of creating delicious and voluminous dinners with ease. With these options, you'll discover that one-pan meals can be both a culinary delight and a practical solution for a satisfying dinner experience.

Grilled and Roasted Delicacies

Ignite your taste buds with the smoky allure of grilled and roasted delicacies that bring a depth of flavor to your dinner table. From succulent meats to perfectly charred vegetables, these recipes showcase the artistry of grilling and roasting, creating dinners that are not only mouthwatering but also in harmony with the principles of the Volumetrics Diet.

1. Balsamic Glazed Grilled Chicken Thighs:

Elevate your dinner with the rich flavors of Balsamic Glazed Grilled Chicken Thighs. Marinate chicken thighs in a balsamic glaze, then grill to perfection. The result is juicy, flavorful chicken with a caramelized exterior, creating a delectable and satisfying main course.

2. Herb-Crusted Grilled Salmon Steaks:

Savor the ocean's bounty with Herb-Crusted Grilled Salmon Steaks. Coat salmon steaks with a medley of fresh herbs and grill to achieve a delightful crust. This grilled masterpiece not only delivers omega-3 fatty acids but also showcases the perfect balance of herbs and char for a dinner that's both nutritious and full of flavor.

3. Rosemary Garlic Roasted Lamb Chops:

Indulge in the robust flavors of Rosemary Garlic Roasted Lamb Chops. Marinate lamb chops in a blend of rosemary, garlic, and olive oil, then roast to perfection. The result is tender, aromatic lamb chops that provide a satisfying and sophisticated dinner experience.

4. Lemon Pepper Grilled Shrimp Skewers:

Bring a taste of the coast to your dinner table with Lemon Pepper Grilled Shrimp Skewers. Marinate shrimp in a zesty lemon pepper seasoning, then thread them onto skewers and grill to perfection. These succulent and flavorful shrimp skewers offer a light yet satisfying option for a delicious dinner.

5. Garlic and Herb Roasted Vegetables:

Elevate your vegetable game with Garlic and Herb Roasted Vegetables. Toss a mix of colorful vegetables, such as bell peppers, carrots, and zucchini, with garlic and herbs, then roast until caramelized. This side dish not only adds vibrancy to your plate but also complements any grilled or roasted main course.

6. Grilled Portobello Mushrooms with Balsamic Glaze:

Celebrate the robust flavor of Portobello mushrooms with Grilled Portobello Mushrooms drizzled in balsamic glaze. The grilling process enhances the earthy notes of the mushrooms, creating a satisfying and versatile dish that can be enjoyed as a main course or a flavorful side.

These grilled and roasted delicacies not only make your dinner a culinary adventure but also highlight the natural flavors of high-quality ingredients. Fire up the grill or preheat the oven, and enjoy the sensory experience of creating dinners that are both flavorful and in line with the fulfilling principles of the Volumetrics Diet. With these recipes, you'll discover that grilling and roasting are not just cooking methods but a celebration of taste and texture in every bite.

Vegetarian Delights for Dinner

Embracing a vegetarian lifestyle opens the door to a world of culinary creativity, where vegetables, fruits, grains, and legumes take center stage. Contrary to the misconception that vegetarian meals lack flavor or variety, there is an abundance of delicious and satisfying options that can tantalize the taste buds and leave you craving more. In this exploration of vegetarian delights for dinner, we'll delve into a selection of mouthwatering dishes that not only celebrate the goodness of plant-based ingredients but also showcase the versatility and richness of vegetarian cuisine.

1. Mouthwatering Mushroom Risotto:

Indulge in the creamy comfort of a well-prepared mushroom risotto. Arborio rice, cooked to perfection in a savory vegetable broth, forms the base for this dish. Sautéed mushrooms, garlic, and onions contribute depth of flavor, while a generous splash of white wine adds a touch of sophistication. Finished with Parmesan cheese and fresh herbs, this dish is a true celebration of earthy, umami-rich flavors.

2. Zesty Chickpea and Spinach Curry:

Dive into the vibrant world of Indian cuisine with a hearty chickpea and spinach curry. Chickpeas, simmered in a fragrant blend of tomatoes, onions, garlic, and a medley of spices, create a robust and satisfying dish. Fresh spinach adds a burst of color and nutrition, making this curry both wholesome and delicious. Serve it over steamed basmati rice or with warm naan bread for a complete and satisfying dinner.

3. Stuffed Bell Peppers with Quinoa and Black Beans:

Elevate your dinner table with colorful stuffed bell peppers filled with a wholesome mixture of quinoa, black beans, corn, and spices. Baked to perfection, these stuffed peppers are not only visually appealing but also a delightful combination of textures and flavors. Top them with a dollop of creamy avocado or a drizzle of lime-infused yogurt for a refreshing finish.

4. Caprese Portobello Mushrooms:

Transform the classic Caprese salad into a hearty main course by replacing tomatoes with large, succulent portobello mushrooms. Grill or roast the mushrooms until tender, then top them with fresh mozzarella, cherry tomatoes, and basil. Drizzle with balsamic glaze for a burst of sweetness, and you'll have a sophisticated yet simple dish that effortlessly captures the essence of Italian flavors.

5. Vegetarian Pad Thai:

Transport your taste buds to the bustling streets of Thailand with a vegetarian twist on the beloved Pad Thai. Rice noodles stir-fried with tofu, bean sprouts, peanuts, and a flavorful tamarind-based sauce create a dish that balances sweet, sour, and spicy notes. Garnish with lime wedges and cilantro for a fresh and invigorating dinner experience.

6. Eggplant Parmesan:

Savor the layers of flavor in a classic Eggplant Parmesan. Thick slices of eggplant are coated in breadcrumbs, baked until golden, and then layered with marinara sauce and melted mozzarella. This Italian-inspired dish is a hearty and satisfying alternative to traditional meat-based Parmesan, showcasing the versatility of eggplant in the culinary world.

7. Quinoa-Stuffed Acorn Squash:

Celebrate the bounty of autumn with quinoa-stuffed acorn squash. Roasted until tender, the acorn squash halves become a vessel for a delectable stuffing made with quinoa, cranberries, pecans, and aromatic spices. This dish not only delights the senses with its vibrant colors but also offers a perfect balance of sweet and savory flavors.

These vegetarian dinner favorites prove that a meatless meal can be anything but mundane. Whether you're a committed vegetarian or simply looking to incorporate more plant-based options into your diet, these delightful recipes are sure to make your dinner table a haven of flavor, nutrition, and satisfaction. So, embrace the abundance of vegetarian delights and let your taste buds embark on a journey of culinary joy.

Chapter 6: Smart Snacks and Desserts

Indulging in smart snacks and desserts doesn't have to compromise your commitment to a healthy and satisfying lifestyle. In this chapter, we'll explore a variety of snacks and desserts that not only cater to your sweet or savory cravings but also align with the principles of the Volumetrics Diet. From guilt-free treats to clever snack choices, these recipes are designed to make your snacking and dessert experiences both enjoyable and fulfilling.

Wholesome and Nutrient-Packed Snacks:

Snacking smartly involves choosing options that not only taste delicious but also contribute to your overall well-being. Let's explore a variety of wholesome and nutrient-packed snacks that provide the perfect balance of flavor and fulfillment.

Guilt-Free Dessert Delights:

Satisfying your sweet tooth doesn't have to derail your health goals. Discover guilt-free dessert delights that use smart ingredient choices to create decadent treats without compromising on nutrition. From fruity creations to chocolatey indulgences, these desserts offer a satisfying conclusion to your meals.

Energy-Boosting Smoothie Bowls:

Give your energy levels a lift with vibrant and nutrient-dense smoothie bowls. Packed with a variety of fruits, vegetables, and wholesome toppings, these bowls not only provide a refreshing snack but also contribute to your daily intake of essential nutrients.

Nourishing Yogurt Parfaits:

Transform your yogurt into a delightful and nourishing parfait. Layered with fresh fruits, granola, and a drizzle of honey, these yogurt parfaits offer a combination of textures and flavors that make for a satisfying and visually appealing snack or dessert.

Baked Goodies with a Healthy Twist:

Enjoy the comforting taste of baked goodies with a healthy twist. Discover recipes that use smart substitutions and portion control to create muffins, cookies, and bars that satisfy your dessert cravings without sacrificing your commitment to a balanced and fulfilling lifestyle.

Savvy Snacking with Nut and Seed Mixes:

Elevate your snacking game with savvy nut and seed mixes that provide a satisfying crunch while delivering a dose of essential nutrients. Explore a variety of combinations that cater to your taste preferences and keep you fueled throughout the day.

Whether you're reaching for a smart snack to curb your midday cravings or treating yourself to a guilt-free dessert after dinner, these recipes in the Smart

Snacks and Desserts chapter will enhance your culinary repertoire. With a focus on ingredients that align with the principles of the Volumetrics Diet, these snacks and desserts will not only satisfy your taste buds but also contribute to your overall sense of well-being. Get ready to enjoy the art of smart indulgence!

Nutrient-Rich Snack Options

Elevate your snacking experience with nutrient-rich options that not only satisfy your cravings but also contribute to your overall well-being. These snacks are designed to be both delicious and fulfilling, aligning with the principles of the Volumetrics Diet.

1. Crunchy Veggie Sticks with Hummus:

Satisfy your snack cravings with a delightful combination of Crunchy Veggie Sticks and Hummus. Slice carrots, cucumber, and bell peppers into sticks for a colorful and nutrient-packed snack. Pair them with a generous serving of hummus for a protein-rich dip that adds flavor and satiety.

2. Greek Yogurt Parfait with Fresh Berries:

Transform your snack routine with a Greek Yogurt Parfait featuring Fresh Berries. Layer high-protein Greek yogurt with a mix of vibrant berries, granola, and a drizzle of honey. This parfait not only satisfies your sweet tooth but also provides a balanced combination of protein, fiber, and antioxidants.

3. Nut and Seed Trail Mix:

Create a Nut and Seed Trail Mix that combines the wholesome goodness of nuts and seeds. Mix almonds, walnuts, pumpkin seeds, and sunflower seeds for a crunchy and nutrient-rich snack. Customize with a touch of dried fruit for a hint of natural sweetness.

4. Sliced Apple with Almond Butter:

Enjoy the classic pairing of Sliced Apple with Almond Butter for a snack that's both satisfying and wholesome. The crispness of apple slices combined with the creamy richness of almond butter creates a delightful combination of textures and flavors, offering a dose of fiber and healthy fats.

5. Edamame and Sea Salt:

Elevate your snacking with Edamame sprinkled with sea salt. These young soybeans are not only a good source of protein but also provide a satisfying crunch. Enjoy them as a savory and nutrient-rich snack that keeps you fueled between meals.

6. Cottage Cheese with Pineapple Chunks:

Turn cottage cheese into a tasty and protein-packed snack by pairing it with Pineapple Chunks. The sweetness of the pineapple complements the creamy texture of cottage cheese, creating a satisfying snack that's rich in protein and vitamin C.

These nutrient-rich snack options not only tantalize your taste buds but also contribute to your daily intake of essential nutrients. Feel free to mix and match these snacks based on your preferences, and discover the joy of incorporating nutrient-packed options into your snacking routine. With these choices, you'll find that smart snacking can be both flavorful and nourishing, enhancing your commitment to a healthy and fulfilling lifestyle.

Guilt-Free Desserts for Sweet Cravings

Satisfy your sweet cravings without compromising your commitment to a healthy lifestyle with guilt-free desserts that are as delicious as they are nutritious. These recipes in the Smart Snacks and Desserts chapter are designed to make your dessert experiences both delightful and aligned with the principles of the Volumetrics Diet.

1. Berry Bliss Frozen Yogurt Popsicles:
Cool down your sweet cravings with Berry Bliss Frozen Yogurt Popsicles. Blend together your favorite berries with Greek yogurt, pour into popsicle molds, and freeze for a refreshing and guilt-free dessert. These popsicles are not only high in antioxidants but also a delightful treat for warmer days.

2. Dark Chocolate-Dipped Strawberries:

Indulge in the classic combination of Dark Chocolate-Dipped Strawberries for a sweet and satisfying dessert. Dip fresh strawberries into melted dark chocolate and let them cool for a delightful treat that not only satisfies your sweet tooth but also provides antioxidants and a touch of decadence.

3. Chia Seed Pudding with Mango Puree:

Create a nutrient-packed dessert with Chia Seed Pudding topped with Mango Puree. Combine chia seeds with your choice of milk and let it set, then layer with a luscious mango puree. This dessert not only offers a delightful texture but also provides a dose of omega-3 fatty acids and fiber.

4. Baked Cinnamon Apple Slices:

Experience the warmth of Baked Cinnamon Apple Slices for a dessert that's comforting and guilt-free. Slice apples, sprinkle with cinnamon, and bake until tender. This simple and wholesome dessert is not only a delicious way to enjoy apples but also adds a touch of sweetness without added sugars.

5. Yogurt and Mixed Berry Parfait:

Delight in a Yogurt and Mixed Berry Parfait that combines the creaminess of yogurt with the sweetness of mixed berries. Layer Greek yogurt with a mix of fresh berries and a sprinkle of granola for a dessert that's both visually appealing and satisfying.

6. Banana Chocolate Chip Oat Cookies:

Indulge in guilt-free Banana Chocolate Chip Oat Cookies that are naturally sweetened and packed with wholesome ingredients. Mash ripe bananas, mix with oats and dark chocolate chips, then bake for a satisfying dessert that's both chewy and nutritious.

These guilt-free desserts for sweet cravings not only cater to your desire for something sweet but also ensure that you enjoy the flavors and textures of delightful treats without compromising on your health goals. Experiment with these recipes, customize them to your liking, and embrace the joy of guilt-free desserts that align with the principles of the Volumetrics Diet. Get ready to satisfy your sweet tooth with treats that are as smart as they are delicious.

Creative Snack Combos for Anytime Munching

Elevate your snacking game with creative combinations that cater to any craving and any time of day. These snack combos are designed to be both satisfying and nutritious, aligning seamlessly with the principles of the Volumetrics Diet. Whether you're looking for a quick energy boost or a flavorful treat, these creative snack ideas have got you covered.

1. Apple Slices with Almond Butter and Granola:

Combine the crispness of apple slices with the creaminess of almond butter and the crunch of granola for a snack that's both satisfying and nutritious. This creative combo offers a balance of fiber, healthy fats, and a touch of sweetness.

2. Cottage Cheese and Pineapple Skewers:

Transform your snack time with Cottage Cheese and Pineapple Skewers. Thread chunks of pineapple and cottage cheese onto skewers for a protein-packed and refreshing snack that satisfies both sweet and savory cravings.

3. Greek Yogurt and Nut Mix Parfait:

Layer Greek yogurt with a mix of nuts and seeds for a parfait that's not only visually appealing but also rich in protein and healthy fats. Customize with your favorite nuts and seeds for a snack combo that keeps you fueled.

4. Avocado and Tomato Salsa Rice Cakes:

Upgrade your rice cake game with Avocado and Tomato Salsa. Spread mashed avocado on rice cakes and top with a flavorful tomato salsa for a satisfying and savory snack that's light yet packed with flavor.

5. Hummus and Veggie Dippers:

Dip into a classic snack combo with Hummus and Veggie Dippers. Slice colorful vegetables like bell peppers, carrots, and cucumbers and pair them with a generous serving of hummus for a crunchy, refreshing, and fiber-rich snack.

6. Turkey and Cheese Roll-Ups with Whole Grain Crackers:
Roll up lean turkey slices and your favorite cheese for a protein-packed snack. Pair these roll-ups with whole grain crackers for a satisfying combination that not only provides energy but also keeps you feeling full.

These creative snack combos are perfect for anytime munching, whether you're looking for a mid-morning pick-me-up, an afternoon treat, or a pre-bedtime snack. Feel free to mix and match these ideas based on your preferences, and discover the joy of smart snacking that aligns with the principles of the Volumetrics Diet. With these combos, you'll have a variety of flavorful and nutritious options to enjoy whenever hunger strikes.

Chapter 7: Crafting Simple Meal Plans

Meal planning is a key element in maintaining a healthy and balanced lifestyle. In this chapter, we'll explore the art of crafting simple meal plans that not only align with the principles of the Volumetrics Diet but also make your journey towards a healthier lifestyle more achievable. Whether you're a seasoned meal planner or a beginner, these tips and sample meal plans will guide you in creating nourishing and satisfying meals throughout your day.

Understanding Portion Control:

Begin your journey into crafting simple meal plans by understanding the importance of portion control. Learn how to balance your meals with the right mix of macronutrients, ensuring that each plate is both satisfying and aligned with your health goals. Discover practical tips for measuring portions and creating a mindful eating experience.

Building Balanced Plates:

Explore the art of building balanced plates that encompass a variety of food groups. From lean proteins and whole grains to colorful vegetables and healthy fats, discover how to create meals that are not only visually appealing but also provide a diverse array of nutrients. Sample plate combinations will serve as inspiration for crafting your own balanced meals.

Incorporating Volumetrics Principles:

Dive into the core principles of the Volumetrics Diet and learn how to incorporate them into your meal plans. Discover the art of choosing high-volume, low-calorie foods that keep you feeling full and satisfied. Explore creative ways to add more fruits, vegetables, and fiber to your meals without compromising on flavor.

Simple and Efficient Batch Cooking:

Streamline your meal preparation with simple and efficient batch cooking techniques. Save time and effort by preparing larger quantities of staple ingredients and versatile recipes that can be used across multiple meals. Learn how to create a weekly cooking routine that ensures you always have nourishing options on hand.

Sample Meal Plans for Success:

Unlock the potential of crafting simple meal plans with sample daily and weekly meal plans. These plans will guide you in creating a variety of meals that are easy to prepare, delicious, and in line with the principles of the Volumetrics Diet. Customize these samples to suit your preferences, making meal planning a personalized and enjoyable part of your routine.

Snack Strategies for Success:

Enhance your meal plans with smart snacking strategies. Learn how to incorporate nutrient-rich snacks between meals to keep your energy levels stable and cravings at bay. Discover a variety of snack ideas that align with the principles of the Volumetrics Diet, ensuring that your snacking is both satisfying and mindful.

Crafting simple meal plans is a powerful tool on your journey to a healthier lifestyle. Whether you're aiming for weight loss, improved well-being, or simply a more balanced diet, the principles and tips in this chapter will guide you in creating meal plans that are practical, enjoyable, and tailored to your individual needs. Get ready to embark on a delicious and fulfilling meal planning adventure!

Weekly Meal Planning Strategies

Master the art of weekly meal planning with strategies that streamline your preparation, enhance efficiency, and ensure a week filled with delicious and balanced meals. These practical tips will guide you in creating a weekly meal plan that aligns seamlessly with the principles of the Volumetrics Diet.

1. Set a Weekly Meal Planning Day:

Choose a specific day each week to dedicate to meal planning. This allows you to take stock of ingredients, plan your meals, and create a shopping list. Consistency in scheduling your meal planning day helps establish a routine and reduces last-minute decision-making.

2. Create a Master List of Go-To Recipes:

Compile a master list of your favorite Volumetrics-friendly recipes. These can be quick and easy meals that you enjoy and that align with your health goals. Having a go-to list simplifies the planning process, allowing you to rotate through meals without feeling overwhelmed.

3. Plan for Variety:

Ensure a diverse and exciting week by incorporating variety into your meal plan. Aim to include a mix of protein sources, whole grains, colorful vegetables, and healthy fats. Variety not only makes your meals more enjoyable but also ensures you receive a wide range of nutrients.

4. Prep Ingredients Ahead of Time:

Save time during the week by prepping certain ingredients ahead of time. Wash and chop vegetables, marinate proteins, and cook grains in bulk. Having these prepared ingredients on hand makes assembling meals quicker and more convenient, especially on busy days.

5. Embrace Theme Nights:

Simplify your decision-making process by incorporating theme nights into your weekly meal plan. For example, designate a specific night for a vegetarian meal, a sheet pan dinner, or a stir-fry. Themes add structure to your plan and make it easier to choose recipes.

6. Plan for Leftovers:

Maximize efficiency by planning for leftovers. Cook larger batches of meals that can be enjoyed for lunch or dinner the next day. This not only saves time but also ensures you have nutritious options readily available.

7. Stay Flexible with Quick Options:

Recognize that life can be unpredictable, and there will be days when your original plan may need to change. Keep a list of quick and simple meals that require minimal preparation for those busy or unexpected days. This ensures you always have a backup plan that aligns with your goals.

8. Use a Meal Planning Template:

Consider using a meal planning template to organize your weekly plan. Whether it's a digital app, a printable template, or a simple notepad, having a structured format helps you stay organized, track your meals, and create a visual guide for the week ahead.

By incorporating these weekly meal planning strategies into your routine, you'll find that creating balanced and satisfying meals becomes a seamless and enjoyable process. Embrace the flexibility of these strategies, and discover the joy of consistently crafting meal plans that align with your health and well-being goals.

Balancing Macros with Volumetrics

Achieving a harmonious balance of macronutrients (macros) is key to crafting meal plans that not only support your health goals but also adhere to the principles of the Volumetrics Diet. In this section, we'll explore the art of balancing proteins, carbohydrates, and fats within the framework of voluminous and satisfying meals.

1. Prioritize Lean Proteins:

Incorporate lean protein sources into your meals to enhance satiety and support muscle health. Opt for options such as grilled chicken, turkey, tofu, beans, lentils, and fish. Balancing your meals with protein-rich foods ensures a steady release of energy and contributes to the feeling of fullness.

2. Embrace Whole Grains:

Choose whole grains as your primary source of carbohydrates to provide sustained energy and essential nutrients. Include options like brown rice, quinoa, whole wheat pasta, and oats. Whole grains contribute to the voluminous nature of meals, promoting a feeling of satisfaction without excessive calories.

3. Prioritize Healthy Fats:

Incorporate healthy fats into your meal plans to support overall well-being. Choose sources like avocados, nuts, seeds, and olive oil. These fats add flavor and richness to your meals, enhancing the sensory experience while contributing to the feeling of fullness.

4. Amplify Veggies and Fruits:

Bulk up your meals with an abundance of vegetables and fruits. These low-calorie, high-volume foods not only contribute essential vitamins and minerals but also add texture and color to your plate. Aim to make half of your plate filled with a variety of colorful and nutrient-dense vegetables.

5. Be Mindful of Portion Sizes:

While volumetrics emphasizes the importance of eating high-volume, low-calorie foods, it's essential to be mindful of overall portion sizes. Balancing macros involves ensuring that your protein, carbohydrate, and fat portions align with your individual dietary needs and goals.

6. Experiment with Balanced Meal Combinations:

Get creative with balanced meal combinations that incorporate all macros in a satisfying manner. For example, a grilled chicken salad with quinoa and a variety of vegetables offers a balanced mix of proteins, carbs, and fats. Experiment with different combinations to find what works best for your taste preferences and nutritional requirements.

7. Use the Volumetrics Principle in Cooking:

Apply the volumetrics principle to cooking techniques. Opt for methods like roasting, grilling, or steaming to enhance the flavors and textures of your ingredients without excess calories. These cooking techniques contribute to the overall voluminous nature of your meals.

8. Stay Hydrated:

Don't forget the importance of staying hydrated throughout the day. Water not only supports overall health but also contributes to the feeling of fullness. Consider incorporating hydrating foods like soups, broths, and water-rich fruits and vegetables into your meal plans.

Balancing macros with volumetrics creates a powerful synergy, allowing you to enjoy satisfying and nutrient-rich meals that contribute to your overall well-being. By prioritizing lean proteins, whole grains, healthy fats, and an abundance of fruits and vegetables, you'll find that crafting balanced meal plans becomes an enjoyable and sustainable part of your healthy lifestyle journey.

Tailoring Meal Plans to Your Lifestyle

One of the keys to successful and sustainable meal planning is tailoring your plans to suit your unique lifestyle. In this section, we'll explore how to craft meal plans that seamlessly integrate into your daily routine, making healthy eating not just a goal but a natural part of your lifestyle.

1. Assess Your Schedule:

Begin by assessing your weekly schedule. Take note of busy days, meetings, and any potential obstacles that might impact your meal preparation time. This evaluation allows you to plan simpler meals or batch cooking on hectic days and more elaborate dishes when you have additional time.

2. Identify Your Cooking Preferences:

Consider your cooking preferences and skills. If you enjoy spending time in the kitchen, you might opt for more intricate recipes. If time is a constraint, focus on quick and easy recipes that require minimal preparation. Aligning your meal plans with your cooking preferences ensures a more enjoyable and sustainable experience.

3. Plan Around Social Commitments:

Take into account social commitments and events when crafting your meal plans. If you have a dinner out planned, adjust your meal plan accordingly. This flexibility allows you to enjoy social occasions without feeling restricted, making your meal plans adaptable to various aspects of your life.

4. Embrace Batch Cooking for Convenience:

If you have a busy lifestyle, embrace the convenience of batch cooking. Prepare larger quantities of key components, such as proteins, grains, and vegetables, during your dedicated meal prep day. This way, you'll have pre-cooked ingredients ready to assemble into quick and nutritious meals throughout the week.

5. Incorporate Grab-and-Go Options:

Include grab-and-go options in your meal plans for days when time is limited. Prepare snack boxes with pre-cut veggies, hummus, and a small serving of nuts or create smoothie packs that can be quickly blended in the morning. Having convenient options ensures you stay on track, even on the busiest days.

6. Tailor Portion Sizes to Your Needs:

Recognize and respect your individual nutritional needs by tailoring portion sizes. Whether you're looking to maintain, lose, or gain weight, adjusting your meal plans to suit your goals ensures that your nutritional intake aligns with your lifestyle and health objectives.

7. Allow Room for Flexibility:

Maintain a level of flexibility in your meal plans to accommodate unexpected events or spontaneous decisions. While planning is essential, being adaptable allows you to navigate deviations without feeling overwhelmed. This approach contributes to a more sustainable and stress-free relationship with meal planning.

8. Make It Enjoyable:

Lastly, ensure that your meal plans bring enjoyment to your life. Incorporate foods you love, experiment with new recipes, and celebrate the culinary journey. When meal planning becomes a source of pleasure, it transforms into a positive and enduring aspect of your lifestyle.

By tailoring your meal plans to your lifestyle, you not only enhance the practicality of healthy eating but also make it a natural and enjoyable part of your daily routine. Whether you're a busy professional, a parent, or someone with a dynamic schedule, personalized meal planning ensures that your dietary choices align seamlessly with the unique aspects of your life.

Conclusion

As we reach the conclusion of the Complete Volumetrics Diet Cookbook, it's time to reflect on the journey of exploring 100+ delicious and satisfying recipes designed to support your health and well-being. This cookbook isn't just a collection of recipes; it's a guide to crafting a healthier lifestyle through the principles of the Volumetrics Diet.

We began by understanding the foundations of the Volumetrics Diet, delving into the science behind it and uncovering the benefits it offers for weight loss and overall health. From there, we ventured into practical aspects, discovering essential tools, ingredients, and smart grocery shopping strategies to set the stage for success.

Our culinary exploration took us through energizing morning smoothies and wholesome oat-based creations for breakfast, followed by protein-packed breakfast bowls that kick-start your day on a satisfying note. For lunch, we embraced fresh and filling salads, hearty soups, and quick and easy lunch wraps, ensuring that midday meals are both nourishing and delightful.

As the day transitioned into evening, our journey continued with flavorful dinner favorites. We explored satisfying one-pan meals that simplify cleanup and grilled and roasted delicacies that celebrate the artistry of cooking. Vegetarian delights showcased the richness of plant-based cuisine, proving that wholesome and delicious dinners don't necessarily require meat.

Our exploration extended into the realm of smart snacks and desserts, where guilt-free treats and creative combinations redefined the concept of indulgence. Nutrient-rich snack options, guilt-free desserts, and energy-boosting smoothie bowls became staples in our repertoire, offering smart choices for any craving or occasion.

Finally, we delved into the practical aspects of crafting simple meal plans, understanding the importance of balancing macros within the voluminous principles of the diet. Weekly meal planning strategies, tailoring meal plans to individual lifestyles, and the joy of experimenting with a variety of recipes provided a roadmap for integrating healthy eating seamlessly into daily life.

As you embark on your culinary journey with the Complete Volumetrics Diet Cookbook, remember that each recipe is a step towards a healthier, more vibrant you. Whether you're seeking weight loss, improved well-being, or simply a more balanced diet, these recipes offer a palette of flavors and textures designed to delight your senses while supporting your health goals.

May these recipes become a source of inspiration in your kitchen, guiding you towards a lifestyle where nutritious and satisfying meals are not just a necessity but a joyful celebration of well-being. Embrace the principles of the Volumetrics Diet, savor each bite, and revel in the transformative power of conscious and fulfilling eating.

Here's to a healthier, happier, and more flavorful you!